UNDESCENDED TESTICLE

PERFECTLY DEALING WITH THE CAUSES OF
UNDESCENDED TESTICLE

DR. AHMED .R

Contents

CHAPTER ONE

INTRODUCTION

A testicle that hasn't shifted into its correct location in the pouch of skin that hangs below the penis (scrotum) before birth is known as an undescended testicle, or cryptorchidism. Usually just one testicle is impacted, however in 10% of cases, neither testicle descends.

In general, undescended testicles are rare, however they are somewhat common in prematurely born boys.

During the first several months of life, the undescended testicle usually finds its right position on its own. Surgery can move your son's undescended testicle into the scrotum if it doesn't straighten out on its own.

Symptoms

The primary indicator that a testicle is undescended is the inability to see or feel it where one would normally find it in the scrotum.

During fetal development, the abdomen is where testicles form. The testicles gradually descend from the abdomen into the scrotum during the final few months of a typical fetal development. This tunnel, known as the inguinal canal, is located in the groin. The process either halts or is slowed down when a testicle is not descended.

Most often, an undescended testicle is found during a postpartum examination of your infant. Find out from the doctor how often your son will need to be checked if he has an undescended testicle. By the time your son is 4 months old, if the testicle hasn't gone into the scrotum, the issue most likely won't go away on its own.

Treating your son's undescended testicle while he is still a baby will help reduce the chance of issues like testicular cancer and infertility later in life.

Boys who are older and have typically descended testicles from birth, ranging from newborns to pre-adolescent boys, may later appear to be "missing" a testicle. This circumstance could suggest:

During a physical examination, a retractile testicle that oscillates between the groin and the scrotum can be easily directed into the scrotum by hand. This is caused by a scrotal muscle reaction and is not abnormal.

An ascending testicle, also known as an acquired undescended testicle, is one that has "returned" to the groin and is difficult to maneuver into the scrotum with the hand.

Speak with your son's physician if you observe any changes in his genitalia or have concerns about his growth.

Unknown is the precise reason of an undescended testicle. Hormones, physical changes, and nerve activity that affect testicular development may be disrupted by a trifecta of genetic, environmental, and maternal variables.

RISK ELEMENTS

A newborn's chance of having an undescended testicle could be heightened by the following factors:

low birth weight

early birth

Undescended testicles in the family or other issues with genital development

Fetal conditions that can limit growth include Down syndrome and defects of the abdominal wall

The mother's use of alcohol during her pregnancy

Mother's cigarette smoking or being around secondhand smoke

Mother's obesity

Type 1 diabetes, type 2 diabetes, or gestational diabetes in mothers

Exposure of parents to specific pesticides

Testicles require a temperature that is marginally lower than the average body temperature in order to mature and operate normally. This colder climate is provided by the scrotum. A boy's testicles continue to change until he is 3 or 4 years old, which has an impact on how well they function later in life.

The following complications can arise from a testicle not being in its proper location:

carcinoma of the testicles. The cells in the testicle that generate immature sperm are typically where testicular cancer starts. It is uncertain what triggers these cells to turn into cancer. Testicular cancer is more common in men who have had an undescended testicle. Testicles in the belly that have not descended are more vulnerable than those in the groin. The risk of testicular cancer in the future may be reduced, but not completely eliminated, by surgically resecting an undescended testicle.

issues with fertility. Men who have had an undescended testicle are more prone to experience low sperm counts, poor sperm quality, and impaired fertility. As early as one year of age, a reduction in sperm-producing cells in the testicles has been observed.

The following are additional issues brought on by the testicle's improper location:

Torsion of the testicles. The twisting of the spermatic cord, which is made up of nerves, blood vessels, and a tube that transports semen from the testicle to the penis, is known as testicular torsion. This excruciating ailment stops the testicle's blood supply. The testicle may be lost if it is not treated right away. Ten times as commonly as in normal testicles, testicular torsion happens in undescended testicles.

trauma. A testicle pressed up against the pubic bone in the groin area may suffer harm.

Hernia inguina. A part of the intestines may protrude into the groin if the aperture between the abdomen and the inguinal canal is very slack.

CHAPTER TWO

Getting Ready for Your Consultation

Typically, an undescended testicle is discovered during birth. Your infant son's well-baby visits, or routine exams, will allow your family doctor or pediatrician to keep an eye on his condition.

Make a list of the questions you want to ask your doctor in advance of your visit. Possible inquiries are as follows:

How frequently should I make appointments?

How can I safely check my scrotum at home to see if the undescended testicle has changed?

When is the best time to consult a specialist?

Which testing is my son going to need?

Which course of treatment would you suggest?

Are there any printed materials, such as brochures, available for me to take home? Which websites would you suggest?

Ask as many questions as you like throughout your appointment.

What to anticipate from your physician

Your baby son's groin will be examined by your doctor. A testicle will feel around for its location by gently rubbing against the skin if it isn't in the scrotum. During the examination, your doctor may use warm, soapy water or a lubricant.

Your doctor will try to gently transfer the testicle into the scrotum if they feel it somewhere in the inguinal canal. It might be an undescended testicle if it just slides partially into the scrotum, if it seems to hurt or discomfort, or if it returns to its former position right away. It's most certainly a retractile testicle if it slides into the scrotum with considerable ease and stays there for a time.

By the time your son is 3 or 4 months old, if his testicle hasn't descended or can't be seen, your doctor should refer you to a pediatric surgeon or a pediatric urologist who specializes in treating urinary tract and genital issues in children for additional testing.

Your son's physician might advise surgery to diagnose and perhaps treat an undescended testicle:

an endoscopy. A tiny abdominal incision is made, and a tiny tube with a camera is introduced. To detect an intra-abdominal testicle, a laparoscopy is performed. In certain situations, a second surgery can be required, but in most cases, the doctor can be able to correct the undescended testicle in the same session. On the other hand, a laparoscopy could reveal the absence of a testicle or a tiny amount of inoperable testicular tissue that needs to be removed.

a surgical incision. In certain situations, direct exploration of the abdomen or groin via a bigger incision might be required.

MEDICATIONS AND SUBTLES

Relocating the undescended testicle to its correct position in the scrotum is the aim of treatment. Testicular cancer and infertility are two consequences of an undescended testicle that may be less likely to occur with early treatment (before one year of age).

Operation

The most common method of correcting an undescended testicle is surgery. During an orchiopexy, the surgeon delicately inserts the testicle into the scrotum and sews it there. Either open surgery or a laparoscope can be used for this technique.

The timing of your son's operation will depend on several things, including his health and the potential difficulty of the procedure. Most likely, your surgeon will advise performing the procedure once your baby is between three and six months old but before he is twelve months old. It seems that receiving surgery early reduces the chance of difficulties down the road.

The testicle may occasionally consist of malformed, aberrant, or dead tissue. This testicular tissue will be removed by the surgeon.

During the procedure, the inguinal hernia is corrected if your son also has one connected to the undescended testicle.

Following the procedure, the surgeon will keep an eye on the testicle to make sure it keeps growing, developing, and staying in its right position. Observation could involve:

physical examination

Scrotal ultrasound examination

hormone level tests

therapy with hormones

Human chorionic gonadotropin (HCG) injections are a part of hormone therapy. This hormone may induce the testicle to migrate to the scrotum of your son. Since hormone therapy is far less effective than surgery, it is often not advised.

Alternative therapies

If one or both of your son's testicles are absent or failed to recover following surgery, you may want to look into saline testicular prosthetics for the scrotum, which can be placed in late childhood or adolescence. With these prosthesis, the scrotum seems normal.

Your doctor will refer you to an endocrinologist (a specialist in hormones) to talk about future hormone therapy that may be required to induce puberty and physical maturity if your kid is not showing signs of physical maturity and has fewer than one healthy testicle.

Orchiopexy, the most common surgical method for treating a single descending testicle, has a nearly 100% success rate. After surgery, male fertility is almost normal for those with one undescended testicle; for those with two, it drops to 65%. Testicular cancer can be prevented by surgery, however it is not completely eradicated.

WAY OF LIFE AND DOMESTIC MEDICINE

It's crucial to monitor the testicles' health even following corrective surgery to make sure normal development occurs. Understanding how your son's body is developing will help. Every time you give him a bath or change his diaper, check where his testicles are located.

Discuss your son's testicles with him when he gets older. As you discuss the physical changes he can anticipate during puberty, let him know how he can examine his own testicles. Testicular self-examination will be a crucial ability for the early diagnosis of potential cancers.

Adapting and providing assistance

Your youngster may be self-conscious about his appearance if he is missing one or both testicles. If he has to undress in front of others in gym class, he may be anxious about how he looks in comparison to his friends or classmates. He might find the following coping mechanisms helpful:

Teach your youngster the appropriate vocabulary to discuss the testicles and scrotum.

Describe how the scrotum typically contains two testicles. Explain to him in straightforward language what it means if one or both are absent and that he is still a healthy boy.

Tell him that he is not sick and that he is not going to get sick.

Ask him if he thinks getting a testicular prosthetic would be a good idea.

Assist him in rehearsing an answer for when he gets mocked or asked about the condition.

Purchase for him swimsuits and boxer shorts that fit loosely so that when he plays sports and changes clothes, the condition won't be as obvious.

Watch out for clues that indicate anxiety or shame, such his quitting a sport he used to enjoy.

THE END